Trigger Point Therapy
with the Foam Roller

D1444730

Trigger Point Therapy with the Foam Roller

Self-Treatment Exercises for Muscle Massage, Myofascial Release, Injury Prevention and Physical Rehab

Dr. Karl Knopf & Chris Knopf

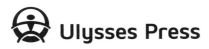 Ulysses Press

Text Copyright © 2014 Karl Knopf. Design and Concept © 2014 Ulysses Press and its licensors. Photographs copyright © 2014 Rapt Productions.

Published in the United States by
Ulysses Press
P.O. Box 3440
Berkeley, CA 94703
www.ulyssespress.com

ISBN: 978-1-61243-354-7
Library of Congress Control Number 2014932311

Printed in Canada by Marquis Book Printing

10 9 8 7 6 5 4 3 2

Acquisitions: Keith Riegert
Managing editor: Claire Chun
Editor: Lily Chou
Proofreader: Lauren Harrison
Indexer: Sayre Van Young
Front cover and interior design: what!design @ whatweb.com
Cover photographs: © Rapt Productions
Interior photographs: © Rapt Productions except on page 15 muscle anatomy © marema/shutterstock.com; page 27 man walking © Viorel Sima/shutterstock.com; page 29 woman high step © Anetlanda/shutterstock.com; page 31 sitting man's back © Stefano Cavoretto/shutterstock.com; page 32 sitting woman's back © Maksim Shmeljov/shutterstock.com; page 33 man's arm and shoulder muscles © Anetta/shutterstock.com; page 34 man with cell © Rido/shutterstock.com; page 35 weightlifter © Ljupco Smokovski/shutterstock.com; page 36 baseball player © Beto Chagas/shutterstock.com; page 37 basketball player © Eugene Onischenko/shutterstock.com; page 38 cyclist © ostill/shutterstock.com; page 39 golfer © tmcphotos/shutterstock.com; page 40 runner © Ariwasabi/shutterstock.com; page 41 soccer player © wavebreakmedia/shutterstock.com; page 42 swimmer © Pavel Sazonov/shutterstock.com; page 43 tennis player © Sveta Orlova/shutterstock.com
Models: Christopher Caruthers, Toni Silver, Nadia Velasquez
Make-up: Sabrina Foster

Distributed by Publishers Group West

Contents

Part 1

Overview

Introduction

To the world you're only one person, but to one person you may be the world! Just like the flight attendant who tells you to put on your own oxygen mask before you help someone else, so it is with you. You can't take care of others until you take care of yourself. And you deserve it!

Today we have good research that shows that when done regularly and performed prudently, simple things such as proper exercise, relaxation and stretching can be used to prevent, alleviate or even restore our bodies to optimal levels. Foam rollers have been used in physical therapy settings for many years. Now they're incorporated in yoga, Pilates and general fitness classes to relax and stretch tight muscles, as well as release tight spots. The foam roller can be used to prevent possible issues and as a rehabilitation tool. Foam rollers with knobs and grooves are especially geared toward releasing trigger points and muscle knots, which can contribute to pain, discomfort and reduced range of motion.

Trigger Point Therapy with the Foam Roller borrows elements from acupressure, massage, and relaxation and flexibility techniques to help you establish normal range of motion, improve flexibility, prevent possible injury and reduce your level of discomfort using the foam roller for trigger point therapy.

Using Foam Rollers for Trigger Point Therapy

Dr. Moshé Feldenkrais is credited for being the first person to use foam rollers for therapeutic purposes (for instance, improving body alignment, reducing muscle tightness and teaching body awareness) in the late 1950s. The beauty of the foam roller is that it can be used by almost everyone. In a therapy setting, foam rollers have been used by clients who have multiple sclerosis as well as those with common orthopedic concerns such as lower back syndrome and rotator cuff issues.

The foam roller is lightweight, easy to use and inexpensive to purchase. It comes in various shapes, sizes and densities and can be purchased online, at sporting goods stores and at physical therapy clinics. The type of foam roller you're probably most familiar with is smooth. The ones this book focuses on are foam rollers with small and large knobs on them to provide a deeper massage than a smooth roller can.

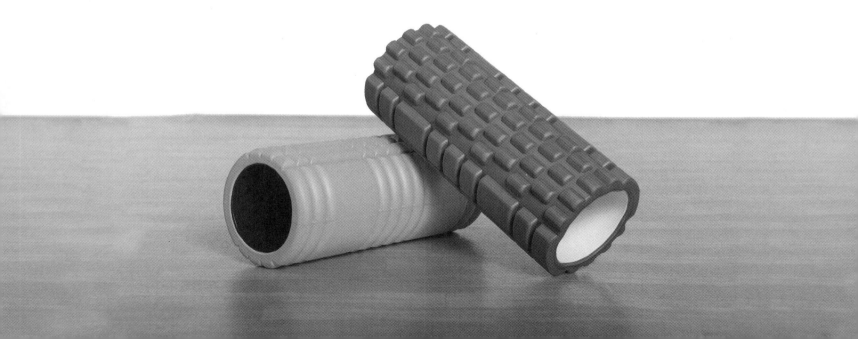

Pain & Self-Myofascial Release

The human body is designed in a remarkable manner and, if well maintained, can function very efficiently for a very long time. However, simply living, combined with chronic missteps and overuse, causes us to sometimes misuse and abuse our bodies, which often leads to poor posture, chronic pain or even disability. Fortunately, we live in a time that offers ample access to both traditional medical treatments as well as complementary options, such as massage, acupressure and biofeedback.

To achieve our fitness goals we often push and hurry. Too often we find that if we don't listen to, observe and use our intuition, nature has a way of getting our attention with an ache or a pain. Pain is our body's warning light, but many of us just disconnect the light and forget about it.

Pain is a major complaint, contributing to about 40 percent of doctor visits. Each of us hurts and feels pain differently—how

we "treat" the pain or discomfort is totally up to us. Many people find relief by using medicines and injections. Others look to complementary options. Unfortunately, sometimes even a combination of these still doesn't result in total relief of chronic discomfort. There's no universal solution—the solution needs to match you and your philosophy.

Understanding pain and discomfort is a complex subject, well beyond the scope of this book. In medicine, doctors can measure our blood pressure and temperature, but measuring pain is very subjective. Some doctors have patients describe their pain using a scale of 1 to 10. Others have patients circle the face that best represents their pain level, like the chart you see below.

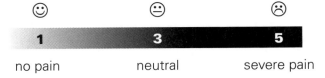

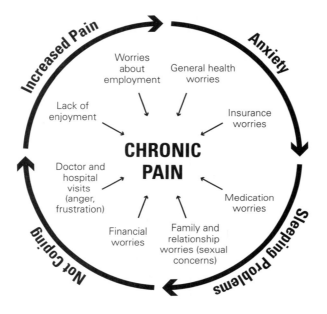

The cycle surrounding CHRONIC PAIN (clockwise): Increased Pain → Anxiety → Sleeping Problems → Not Coping → (back to Increased Pain)

Worries about employment, General health worries, Insurance worries, Medication worries, Family and relationship worries (sexual concerns), Financial worries, Doctor and hospital visits (anger, frustration), Lack of enjoyment

Research has shown that stretching, relaxation, meditation, trigger point treatments and biofeedback techniques ease muscle tension that contributes to pain. Regular stretching is useful to release muscle tension and lengthen shortened muscles, decreasing pain. Massage is most people's favorite because it can reduce anxiety that contributes to reducing muscle tension. Massage can also increase blood flow to an area, which may hasten healing.

Massage is the manipulation of superficial and deeper layers of muscle and connective tissue using various techniques. Massage is used to enhance function, aid in the healing process, decrease muscle reflex activity, inhibit motor-neuron excitability, and promote relaxation and well-being. Most experts agree on the following benefits of a massage:

- Promotes relaxation, causing a temporary reduction in resting heart rate and blood pressure
- Increases circulation to the area
- Decreases muscle spasms
- Promotes lymph flow
- Improves muscle flexibility
- Decreases scar tissue
- Decreases the sensation of pain
- Fosters relaxation
- Improves posture

It's believed that when soft tissue gets injured (whether through trauma, overtraining or chronic misuse), the thin layer on top of or between muscles (the fascia or myofascia) gets "sticky." If the fascia does not slide freely, muscle stiffness and soreness can result. In addition, some experts suggest that the tight, tender spots we often notice in our muscles can later manifest themselves as a chronic condition if not addressed early on. The concept of trigger point therapy or acupressure is that locating a "tight spot" can release tension of a muscle. Myofascial release techniques are similar in providing the results often gained from acupressure and trigger point treatments. While trigger point treatments, acupressure and the like need to be done by a trained professional, most of us can perform self-myofascial release. Maintaining a good level of soft tissue quality is important in that it can assist you in being flexible and pain free.

Research shows that getting on top of the pain early, before it transforms into chronic discomfort, is wise. Toughing it out might not always be smart, no matter what your coach told you. Acute pain that's controlled early is less likely to become a chronic pain syndrome; it's much more difficult to eliminate established pain.

For any pain, consult your health professional to rule out any serious causes. Pain in one area can be referred from a source far away. For example, pain between the shoulder blades could be a sign of a heart attack, while pain in the calf muscle could be referred from the nerves in your lower back.

Self-myofascial release techniques are designed to release muscle tension brought on by trauma, repetitive use or being overly sedentary. Performing simple self-myofascial release moves daily with the foam roller can keep muscles fluid, prevent future issues and offer many other benefits. Improved blood flow increases the amount of oxygen and nutrients to the area, which can foster improvements.

What Are Trigger Points?

There are approximately 40 muscles in the human body. Due to local trauma to the muscle as a result of overuse, overstretching, deconditioning, injury or illness, trigger points may form in a small number of muscle fibers in a larger muscle or muscle bundle. There are approximately 620 potential trigger points in human muscles, and they reportedly show up in the same places in every person. In an active trigger point, pain can either be local or felt in another location, called referred pain. A latent trigger point is one that exists, but does not yet refer pain. Any muscle can develop an individual trigger point or multiple points. Some of the most common areas are the neck and shoulders, lower back and buttocks.

Latent trigger points can influence muscle activation patterns, which can result in poor muscle coordination and balance. Many people call active and latent trigger points "ouch" points, whereby just pressing on the point elicits pain. (People with fibromyalgia understand this all too well.) When trigger points are present in muscles, there's often pain and weakness in the associated structures. These points can in turn pull on tendons and ligaments associated with the muscle and can cause pain deep within a joint where there are no muscles. The integrated hypothesis theory states that trigger points form from excessive release of acetylcholine, which produces sustained depolarization of muscle fibers.

Today, much treatment of trigger points is administered by massage therapists, physical therapists, osteopathic physicians, occupational therapists, myotherapists, athletic trainers, chiropractors and acupressure practitioners. Practitioners claim to have identified reliable referred-pain patterns that associate pain in one location with trigger points elsewhere. Compression of a trigger point may elicit local tenderness, referred pain or local twitch response.

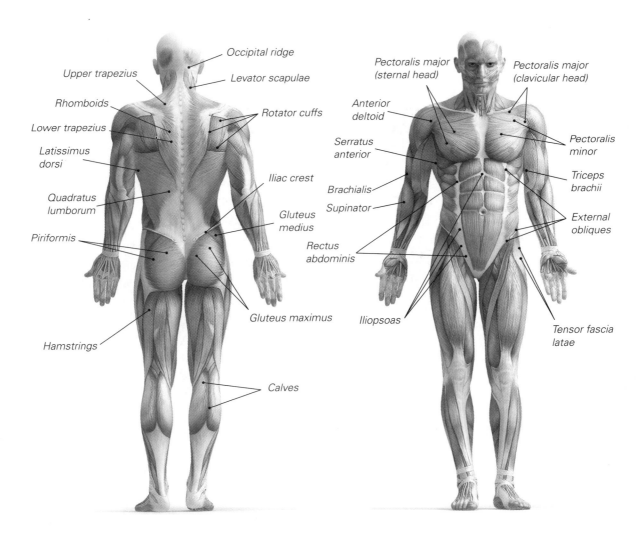

Occipital ridge

Upper trapezius

Levator scapulae

Rhomboids

Rotator cuffs

Lower trapezius

Latissimus dorsi

Quadratus lumborum

Iliac crest

Gluteus medius

Piriformis

Gluteus maximus

Hamstrings

Calves

Pectoralis major (sternal head)

Pectoralis major (clavicular head)

Anterior deltoid

Serratus anterior

Pectoralis minor

Brachialis

Triceps brachii

Supinator

External obliques

Rectus abdominis

Iliopsoas

Tensor fascia latae

COMMON TRIGGER POINTS

What Are Trigger Points?   15

Why Use the Foam Roller for Trigger Point Therapy?

Too often, chronic poor posture and improper body mechanics along with overtraining specific muscles leads to increased muscle tension and muscle imbalances. Additionally, a trauma to an area can also increase muscle tension, which often contributes to muscle spasms. Often as a result of a trauma to an area, a person develops "knots" or "trigger point discomfort."

If these dysfunctions aren't addressed properly, they can lead to reduced mobility and chronic problems. Performing myofascial techniques with a foam roller designed for trigger point therapy along with a systematic stretching routine can facilitate the breakup of these sticky adhesions.

The beauty of the programs in this book is that they can be done as stand-alone routines or performed in conjunction with your regular training regimen, either prior to or after a workout to relax tight muscles. In addition, the movements can be done anywhere, anytime. In any case, they work to break up interwoven muscle fibers to improve blood flow into the muscles. The only requirement of the programs is time on task and being in tune with your body's communication system.

How to Use the Foam Roller for Trigger Point Therapy

The concept behind self-myofascial release methods is to think of yourself as a world-class massage therapist. Good massage therapists don't say, "I'll spend five minutes on your legs and three minutes on your shoulders." Instead, they allow your body to provide them feedback via their hands of where to go and how hard to press. In a similar fashion, you should let your body tell you what it wants. Some days you'll need to spend more time on your upper back while on other days you'll want more time on your legs—just follow your body's suggestions.

Each of us has a different threshold for discomfort and each body part requires different amounts of pressure. Aim for what "hurts so good." Start with a light touch and move to deeper pressure. The legs are often very sensitive, whereas the back, buttocks and shoulders often can tolerate more pressure; exercise caution when performing any releases around the abdominal and neck regions, or any area where you have any health issues. It's okay to press a tight spot until uncomfortable then back off. While some experts suggest holding a spot for long periods of time, this experience is not a test of your pain tolerance! Only hold as long as you can tolerate it. Don't let anyone "should" you! Use your common sense.

To obtain optimal results, tune out external distractions and tune in to your internal communication. The time you spend doing self-massage with the foam roller should be a mindful experience. If you stay mindful to your body's instructions, it will direct you where to place the roller, how much intensity you should place against your body and how long to hold the position. Using the foam roller in combination with mindful breathing can aid in the outcome. A suggested breathing plan is to inhale slowly, either through the nose or mouth fully, for a count of 4 to 6 and then exhale slowly through the lips (as if blowing out a candle) for a count of 8 to 12.

Basically, you need to act as if you're the best massage therapist in world. There's no absolute right way to perform each movement. Some days, significant pressure will feel fine, while on other days the slightest pressure hurts. When doing a self-massage, try to start at the proximal (top) parts of the body or limb. For example, start at the thigh and move toward the foot.

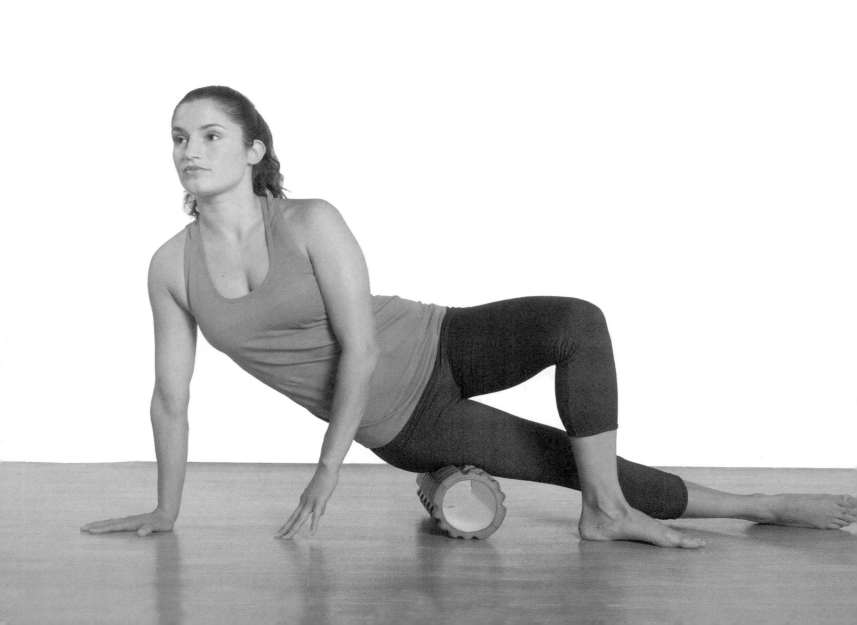

If you feel worse after a session, consider reducing the intensity and/or duration of the session. Remember that self-massage and myofascial-release sessions are not magical cures. If you're experiencing chronic pain, it's imperative that you ascertain the cause by seeking medical advice. Masking pain with a massage is no better than masking your pain with drugs or alcohol.

The key to effective use of foam rollers for trigger point therapy lies in the following concepts:

- Understand how long and how much pressure to apply is correct for you.

- Understand the expected outcomes of the program.

- Be relaxed and warm.

- Dress in clothes that allow you freedom of movement.

- Understand the interconnectedness of how tight hamstrings influence lower back pain. Learn which order of treatment is best for you. Generally, large muscle groups are followed by isolated muscles

- Focus on areas of tension, but don't go beyond mild discomfort. Benefits are not going to come if you're in pain since pain causes tightness. You should feel better when you release.

- Be patient; don't expect overnight results. You don't need to hold the position to a point of pain.

- While self-massage is generally considered safe, it's still wise to be cautious.

- Never massage an area where inflammation or swelling is present.

- Never massage a bony area.

- If you experience soreness that lasts more than 24 hours, re-evaluate the routine. Never do too much too soon.

- Avoid any area that has been injured until cleared by your health provider.

- Speak to your health provider if you're pregnant or have osteoporosis.

- Never self-diagnosis yourself—pain is your body's warning system. Always seek medical advice.

- Seek medical advice if you're in poor health, in severe pain and/or have poor range of motion/flexibility.

- When lying on the foam roller, align your spine correctly.

- Don't focus on duration—use your body as a guide.

- No particular direction is right or wrong.

Foam rollers are a wonderful way to improve mobility and release tension while adding diversity to your standard exercise program. This book encourages you to experiment with duration and intensities that offer you the ideal response. Just remember: If you allow too much time to lapse between sessions, the adhesions reform and you have to start over. A little bit done regularly is far more beneficial than a lot done infrequently.

Before You Begin

While foam roller exercises are considered an acceptable method with which to stretch and perform self-massage, this book isn't intended as a replacement for physical therapy or a trained massage therapist. However, it can be a nice complement as a home-based post-rehab routine or a preventative program.

If you have a pre-existing condition of any kind, consult your health professional about how you can best use the roller.

If you have a chronic injury, use this book in concert with feedback from your health provider or massage therapist to help you develop a better-balanced body.

The moves presented in this book are not intended to "cure" anything. Be careful about executing any positions over spots that provide circulation to an area, bony body parts or joints. Start slowly and experiment with what feels best for you in regards to intensity and duration.

Getting On and Off the Roller

Using a foam roller for trigger point therapy for self–muscle release is easy, but utilizing it correctly is a little tricky at first. Before you roll away your aches and pains, make sure you know how to get on the roller safely and gracefully. Always make sure that the area around you provides you enough space to perform the moves. If getting on the floor is an issue, try placing the roller in the middle of the bed.

Safety Tips
- Use the roller only on non-slip surfaces.
- Avoid applying pressure over joints, bony areas, and internal organs.
- Don't make pain—relax and enjoy.

The trickiest position is probably lying along the length of the roller on your back. To do so, place the roller on the floor or bed. Sit at the end of the roller with your knees bent and feet on the floor, and then slowly lie back on the roller until your head is resting on the roller. The roller will run from your tailbone to your head. To get off the roller, just roll to the side or reverse the process.

To lie facedown on the roller, you'll likely want to start from a kneeling position and either place the roller where needed or roll into the start position.

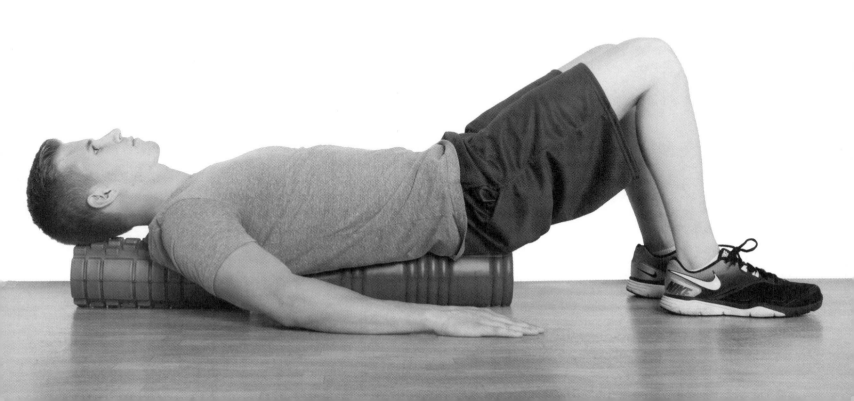

Part 2
Programs

How to Use This Book

This section features several programs that address all the major areas of the body. Detailed instructions on how to perform the movements can be found in Part 3. Feel free to choose one of these programs and perform it as noted, or add any exercises from Part 3 as you see fit. To create your own routine, see "Program Design" on page 26.

Keep in mind that using a foam roller may look like child's play, but utilizing it correctly to obtain an ideal response is no easy feat. If you've been diagnosed with a medical condition, it's highly recommended that you obtain personalized instruction from a trained therapist prior to engaging in any of these programs or exercises. This book should be used in concert with your health provider to assist you to a better-balanced body. Your body, just like a spinning top, functions best when all the forces are in sync.

It's prudent to tune in to your body while engaging in self-massage and be intuitive about positioning and the amount of pressure you exert. Engaging in a relaxation session before or together with these trigger point massages will amplify the experience. There are many methods that can help you relax, including taking a warm bath or applying a heating pad to improve circulation to the area. Some people turn on smoothing music. Consider "centering" yourself prior to any session by doing some slow diaphragmatic breathing: breathe in through your nose for 4 counts, hold for 1 to 2 counts, and exhale through your lips for 4 counts. If you rush through the moves, the results could be less than ideal. If you are doing diaphragmatic breathing properly, your belly will rise when inhaling and drop when exhaling.

As for how long you should roll or hold the position? Do as much or as little as needed. Each body is different. Just keep in mind that none of the hold positions should be painful. Press down until uncomfortable and then back off slightly. Each person will have different pressure tolerance, so a little experimentation is needed. If these moves are done regularly, you're likely to experience less muscle stiffness and a more relaxed state of mind and perhaps even lower your blood pressure.

Program Design

An ancient physician once told his medical students, "If you listen to your patients, they will tell you their cure." So it is with you. If you truly listen to your body, it will tell you which exercises are correct for you. It's very possible that the trigger point massages you select will change daily depending on the demands placed upon you that day. A difficult day sitting over a computer will necessitate a different set of massages than a day of yard work. Another suggestion is to ask your health professional where you're tight, or to look in the mirror—are you hunched over? You're a unique design, so design a program that's unique for you!

You'll see that the movements in this book can be done while sitting in a chair, sitting on the floor, and lying on your stomach (prone) or back (supine) and even on your side. Seated movements are a nice way to acquaint your body with foam roller massages. Starting in a chair allows you better control of the pressure applied to the area. When doing massage from any lying position for the first time, apply the gentlest amount of pressure and adjust as your body instructs you. If you wish, you can rest your head on a pillow.

General Program

This program combined with a regular flexibility program will help you stay limber and relaxed. This program covers common tight spots developed in normal activities of daily living, such as walking and sitting at a desk.

Exercise

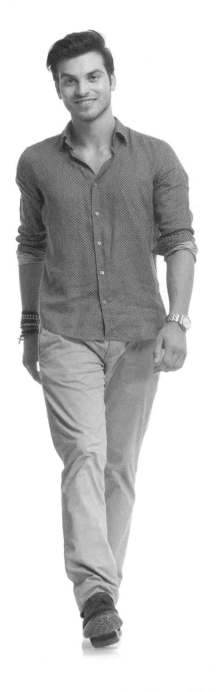

Posture Program

This program is designed to release the muscular tension in your body that often contributes to poor posture. The focal areas of this program are the chest, shoulders, and upper and lower back.

Exercise

Upper & Lower Back Release	page 54
Glute Massage	page 67
Chest Release	page 61
Hip Flexor Release	page 64
Spine Extension	page 66
Neck Release	page 72
Upper Back & Shoulder Massage	page 70
Supine Fly	page 77

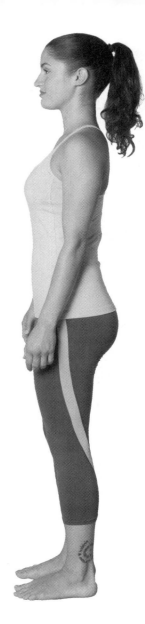

Foot & Leg Release Program

Folks who are very active tend to have tight leg muscles, including the hamstrings (back of thigh), quadriceps (front of thigh) and iliotibial band (side of thigh). People who sit a great deal of the day can also have tight hamstrings, which can contribute to lower back issues. The goal of this program is to balance out these muscles and release tension often found in the legs and feet. Runners and bicyclists who also have sore calves, shins and/or feet should find some relief here.

Exercise

Foot Massage	*page 47*
Ankle & Foot Sequence	*page 48*
Hamstring Release (Chair)	*page 56*
Quad Massage	*page 58*
Hamstring Release	*page 84*
Total Calf Release	*page 83*
Iliotibial Band Release	*page 87*

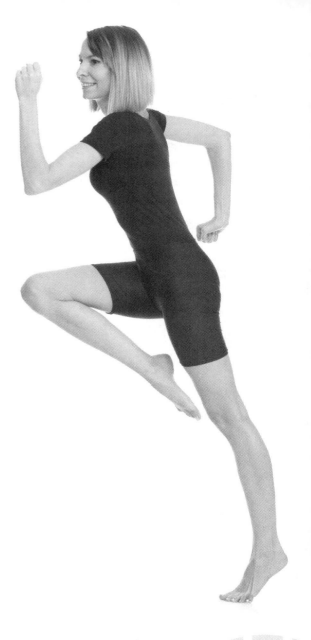

Upper Back Release Program

This program is designed for releasing the upper back. Folks who work long hours over a desk tend to have a prolonged rounded back position, which can contribute to poor posture, as well as a stiff neck and shoulder region. Swimmers and people who do a great deal of chest exercises at the gym also tend to have a rounded upper back. This program should address these issues.

Exercise

Upper & Lower Back Release	*page 54*
Upper Back Release (Seated)	*page 52*
Chest Release	*page 61*
Chest & Shoulder Release	*page 62*
Spine Extension	*page 66*
Neck Release	*page 72*
Upper Back Release	*page 68*
Upper Back & Shoulder Massage	*page 70*

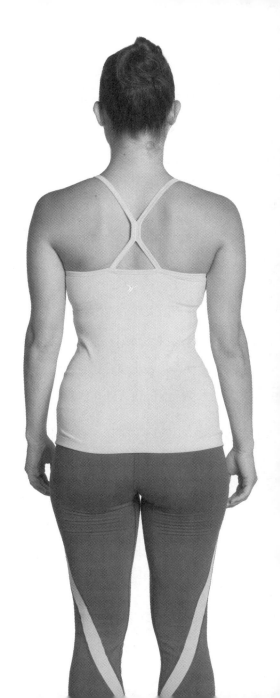

Lower Back Release Program

Most people have a lower back issue at some time in their life. Often the cause is the result of muscle fatigue and tension, whether from sitting or standing all day, lifting heavy objects incorrectly or poor biomechanics in general. This program attempts to focus on the areas of the body that often contribute to lower back stiffness. *Note:* If you're having prolonged back pain or numbness, consult your doctor.

Exercise

Lower Back Release	*page 50*
Mid-Back Release	*page 75*
Lower Back Expansion	*page 76*
Supine Fly	*page 77*
Shoulder Protraction/Retraction	*page 78*
Hip Flexor Extender	*page 79*

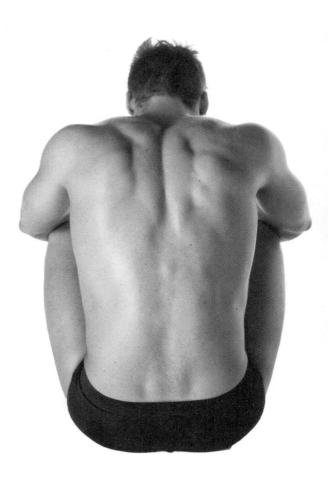

Total Back Release Program

This abbreviated program is aimed at people who know they need to release the muscular tension of their back but don't have time for the separate upper and lower back release programs on pages 30 and 31. *Note:* If you're having prolonged back pain or numbness, consult your doctor.

Exercise

Combo Special	*page 93*
Spine Extension	*page 66*
Upper Back Release	*page 68*
Upper Back & Shoulder Massage	*page 70*
Lower Back Expansion	*page 76*
Supine I's, Y's & T's	*page 80*
Piriformis Release	*page 88*

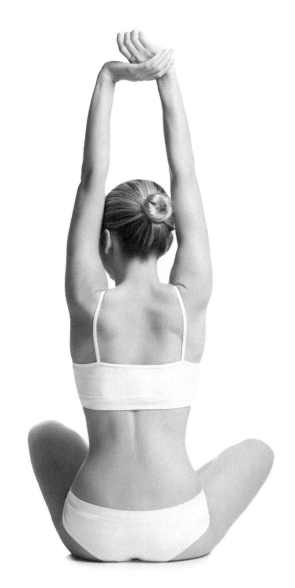

Shoulder & Arm Release Program

This program is designed for people who use their arms and shoulders a great deal in work or play. If you're a baseball/softball player, swimmer, painter or similar, take time to engage in this routine. If you're over 50, be mindful of the moves in this program since many 50-plus folks have shoulder issues.

Exercise

Lat Release	*page 89*
Triceps Massage	*page 90*
Supine I's, Y's & T's	*page 80*
Shoulder Protraction/Retraction	*page 78*
Supine Fly	*page 77*
Biceps Release	*page 63*
Forearm Massage (Seated)	*page 49*
Forearm Massage	*page 57*

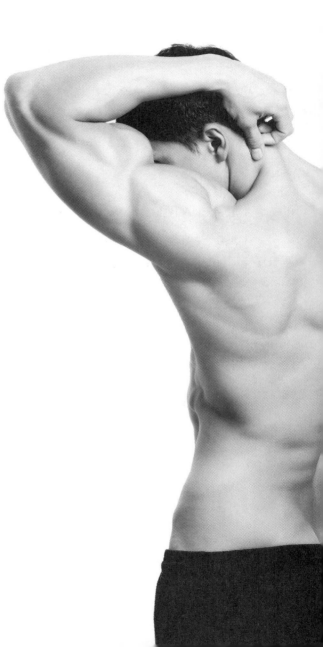

Computer Work Release Program

How many hours do you hunch over a smartphone or a computer, only to go home at night and complain that your back is stiff and sore? Try this routine daily and see if it provides some relief.

Exercise

Upper Back Release (Seated)	page 52
Lower Back Release	page 50
Mid-Back Release	page 75
Chest Expander	page 73
Hip Flexor Release	page 64
Chest & Shoulder Release	page 62

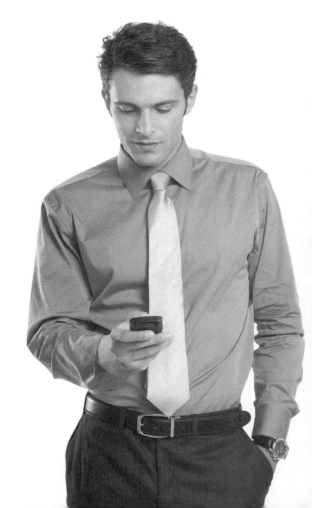

Active Person's Release Program

This program is designed for the all-around active person, from crosstrainer to runner to weightlifter. Treat your body kindly so that it will continue to let you pursue your favorite athletic activities.

Exercise

Quad Stretch	*page 59*
Quad Release	*page 65*
Iliotibial Band Release	*page 87*
Piriformis Release	*page 88*
Total Calf Release	*page 83*
Lower Back Stretch	*page 60*
Chest & Shoulder Release	*page 62*
Upper Back Release	*page 68*
Lat Release	*page 89*

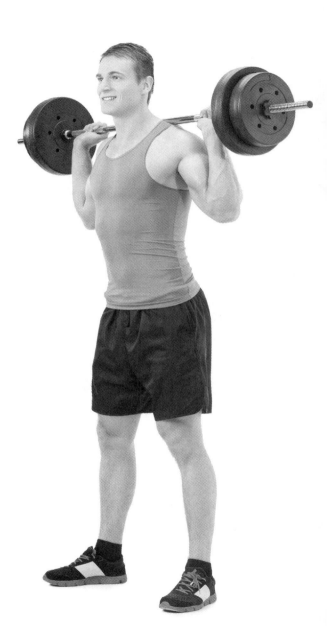

Baseball/Softball Program

People of all ages can play baseball and softball, which can work your legs, arms and shoulders. If you want to be able to swing for the fences and continue running those bases, a regular dose of foam rolling is a good idea.

Exercise

Quad Massage	*page 58*
Hamstring Release	*page 84*
Iliotibial Band Release	*page 87*
Psoas Release	*page 85*
Sacrum Release	*page 86*
Chest & Shoulder Release	*page 62*
Spine Extension	*page 66*
Upper Back Release	*page 68*
Upper Back & Shoulder Massage	*page 70*

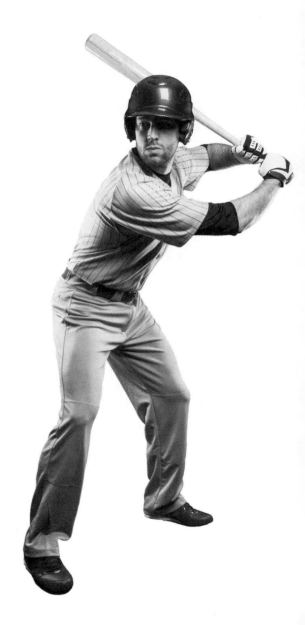

Basketball Program

Basketball is an explosive and jarring sport that uses your legs, chest and shoulders. This program will bring balance to those areas.

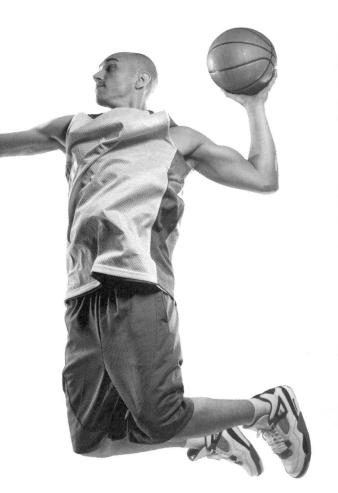

Exercise

Foot Massage	*page 47*
Hamstring Release (Chair)	*page 56*
Quad Stretch	*page 59*
Lower Back Stretch	*page 60*
Chest & Shoulder Release	*page 62*
Upper Back Release	*page 68*
Iliotibial Band Release	*page 87*

Bicycling Program

Biking ostensibly works the lower body and cardiovascular system, but cyclists often acquire a rounded posture from hunching over the handlebars. Foam roller sessions should improve shoulder and chest flexibility, as well as maintain range of motion in the legs.

Exercise

Hamstring Release (Chair)	page 56
Upper Back Release (Seated)	page 52
Quad Stretch	page 59
Lower Back Stretch	page 60
Chest & Shoulder Release	page 62
Upper Back Release	page 68
Supine Fly	page 77
Quad Massage	page 58
Hamstring Release	page 84

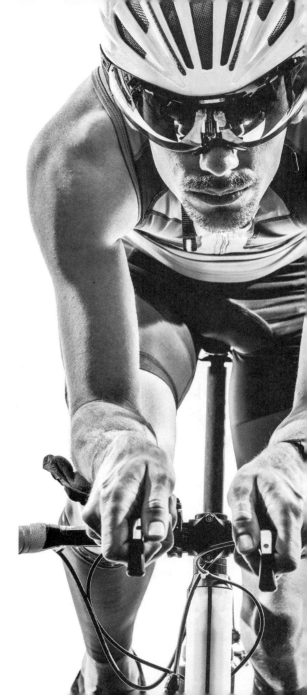

Golf Program

Golf can take a toll on the knees, hips and lower back. Regular foam roller sessions will keep you mobile and swinging.

Exercise

Upper Back Release (Seated)	page 52
Lower Back Release	page 50
Mid-Back Release	page 75
Chest & Shoulder Release	page 62
Lower Back Stretch	page 60
Upper Back & Shoulder Massage	page 70
Supine Fly	page 77

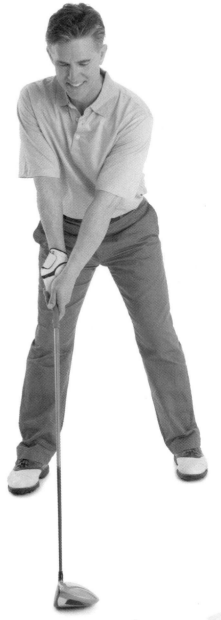

Running/Jogging Program

Runners and joggers invariably experience tight calves, quads and hamstrings. Regular foam roller work can help you stay flexible and injury free.

Exercise

Foot Massage	page 47
Hamstring Release (Chair)	page 56
Quad Stretch	page 59
Lower Back Stretch	page 60
Chest & Shoulder Release	page 62
Upper Back Release	page 68
Iliotibial Band Release	page 87

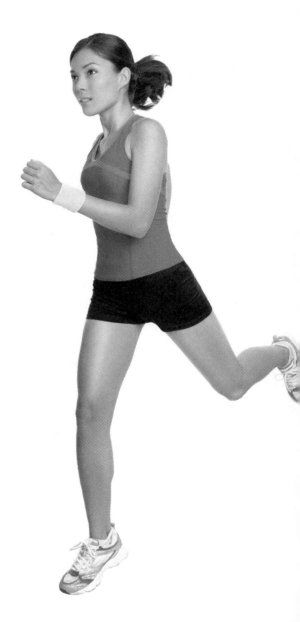

Soccer Program

Soccer is an intense sport that utilizes the quads, hamstrings and calves. Regular foam rolling will help keep you on the field.

Exercise

Hamstring Release (Chair)	*page 56*
Upper Back Release (Seated)	*page 52*
Quad Stretch	*page 59*
Lower Back Stretch	*page 60*
Quad Massage	*page 58*
Hamstring Release	*page 84*
Psoas Release	*page 85*
Sacrum Release	*page 86*

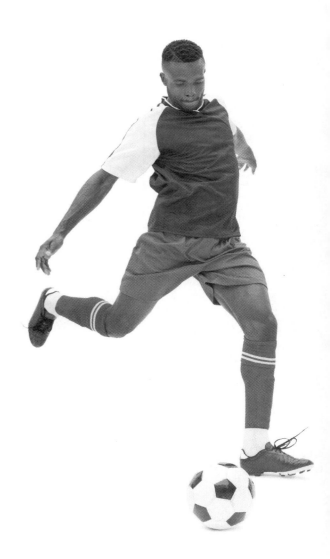

Swimming Program

Swimming is an excellent overall-fitness activity, but swimmers often get a rounded posture. Regular foam roller sessions help to improve shoulder and chest flexibility.

Exercise

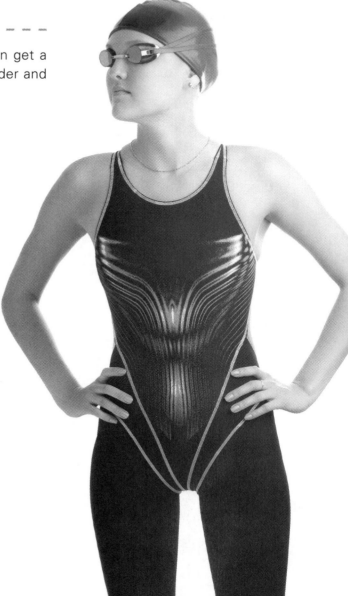

Tennis Program

Tennis is a great full-body workout that works the legs, torso, chest and shoulders. Regular foam roller sessions will help ensure you don't miss a day on the court.

Exercise

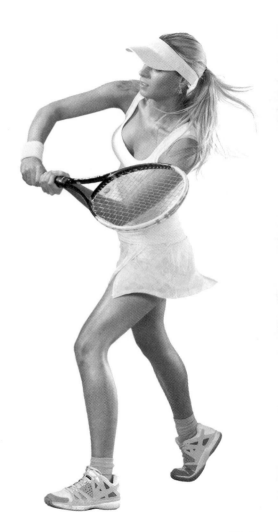

Part 3

Exercises

Foot Massage

This can be performed using one foot or both feet at a time. Make sure you do this movement in a sturdy chair.

Starting Position: While seated, place the roller under one foot.

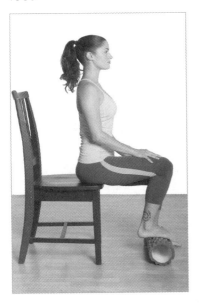

1–2: Apply pressure, rolling and pressing the bottom and sides of your foot over the roller, stopping at tight areas and holding for a few moments. Use your intuition to know how hard to press and how long to hold. Aim to hold the position for 5 to 30 seconds. Relax and repeat as desired. Breathe slowly and fully.

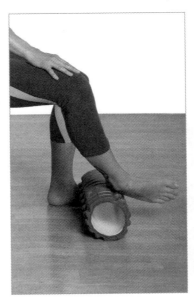
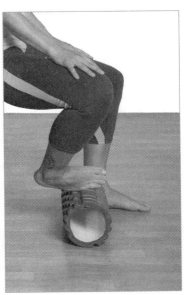

Ankle & Foot Sequence

Starting Position: Sit upright in a chair. Place the roller on the floor and rest your feet on top.

1–2: Slowly and gently roll your ankles forward and back. Remember to stay in your pain-free zone.

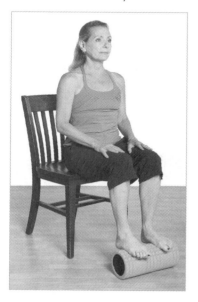

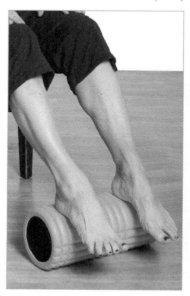

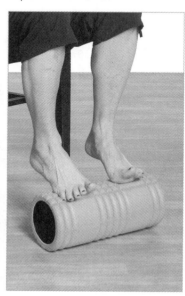

Forearm Massage (Seated)

Starting Position: While seated at a table, rest your forearm (near your wrist) on the roller.

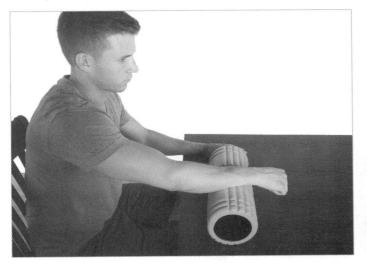

1–2: Roll and press your forearm along the roller, applying the amount of pressure that feels right. It's okay to rotate your arm as you roll. Use your intuition on how hard to press and how long to hold any one position. Hold for 5 to 30 seconds. Breathe slowly and fully.

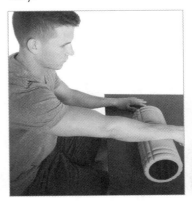 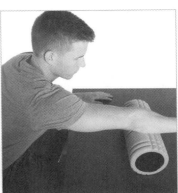

Switch sides.

Lower Back Release

Starting Position: Sit in a chair with a solid high back. Place a short roller in the small of your back.

1: Press your body into the roller, gently and slowly arching your back.

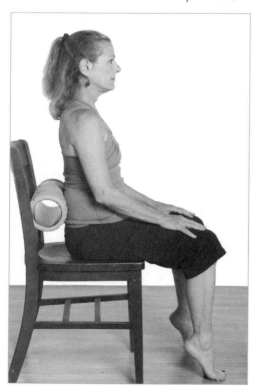
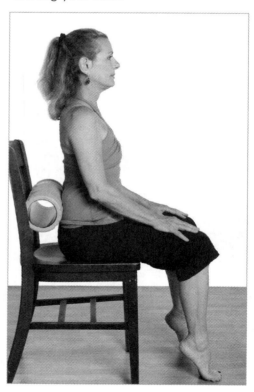

2: Now round your back as much as is comfortable as you press into the roller.

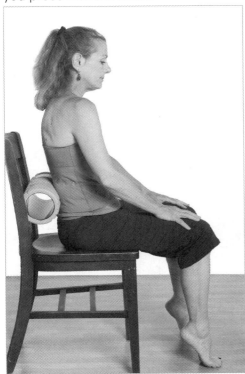

Continue arching, extending and applying pressure where desired. Perform for 5 to 30 seconds.

Upper Back Release (Seated)

Starting Position: Sit in a chair with a solid high back. Place a short roller horizontally just under your shoulder blades.

1: Press your body into the roller, squeezing your shoulder blades together as you hold.

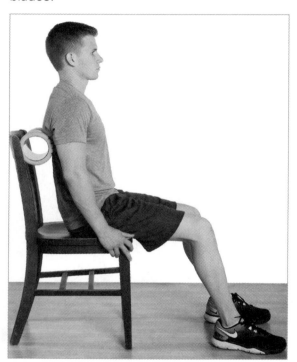

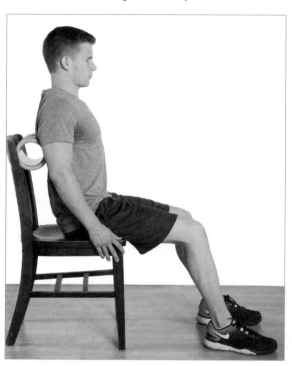

2: Now roll your shoulders forward as you press into the roller.

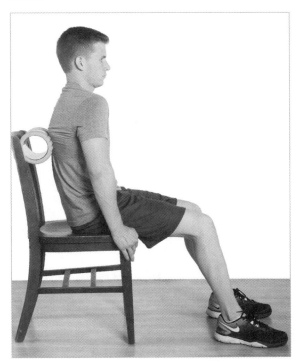

Raise or lower the roller to find your tight spots. Hold for 5 to 30 seconds.

Upper & Lower Back Release

Starting Position: Sit in a chair with a solid high back. Place the roller vertically along the back of the chair and carefully position your spine against it.

1: Press your body into the roller and hold as desired. Hold for 5 to 30 seconds. Breathe slowly and fully.

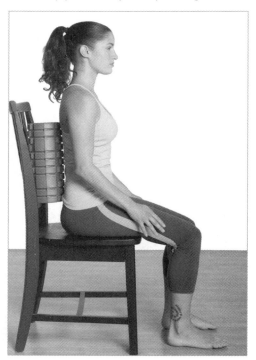

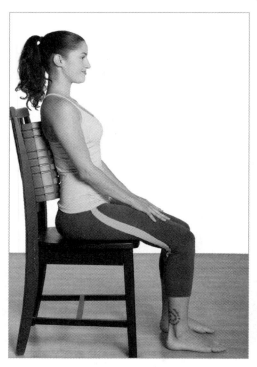

2: Now slowly roll from side to side.

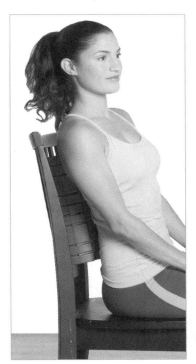
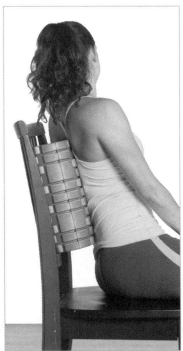

Variation: To better expand your rib cage, inhale while opening your arms out to the sides into a "T" position, then exhale while bringing your arms back in front of your chest.

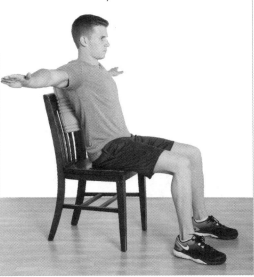

Hamstring Release (Chair)

This can be done with one or both legs at the same time.

Starting Position: Sit in a chair and place the roller under one thigh. Gently roll and press your leg along the roller as desired, returning to any area with particular tension. Hold for 5 to 30 seconds. Breathe slowly and fully.

Modification: This can also be done while sitting on the ground.

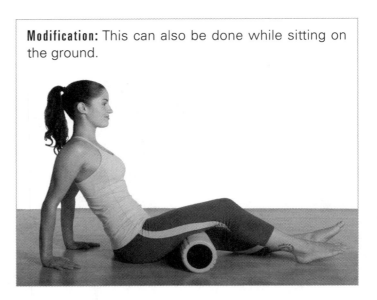

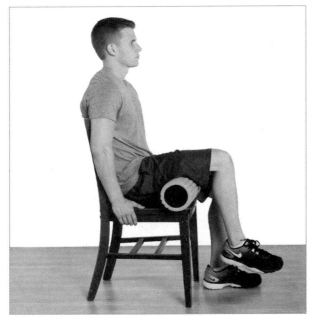

Switch sides.

Forearm Massage

Starting Position: While kneeling with your butt toward your heels, place your wrists on top of the roller, palms down.

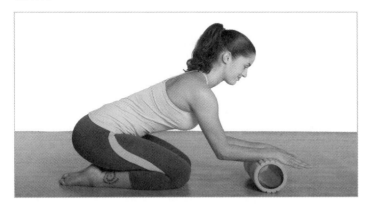

Variation: Rotate your forearm so that your thumb points up to obtain a different angle of release.

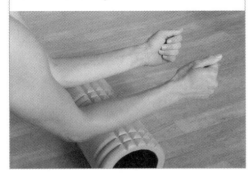

1: Apply the desired amount of pressure and hold.

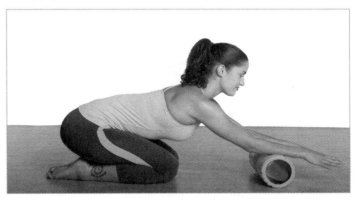

Using your body motion to move you forward and back, roll your forearms along the roller to get a complete forearm massage. Return to any area with particular tension if desired, pressing into the roller. Hold for 5 to 30 seconds. Breathe slowly and fully.

Quad Massage

Starting Position: While kneeling, place the roller against your thighs, just above your knees.

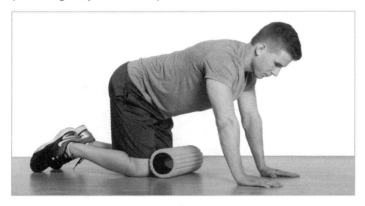

1: Lower onto your hands and gently apply pressure to your thighs.

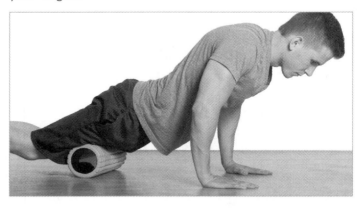

Roll up and down the roller, below your hips and above your knees, stopping at any tight spots. Hold for 5 to 30 seconds.

Quad Stretch

Starting Position: While kneeling, place the roller on your thighs, close to your hip crease.

1–2: Slowly and gradually fold over the roller, reaching forward with your arms. Breathe slowly and fully, letting your muscles relax.

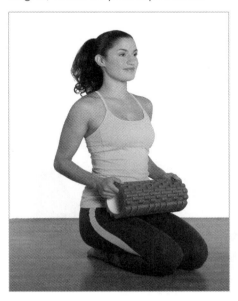

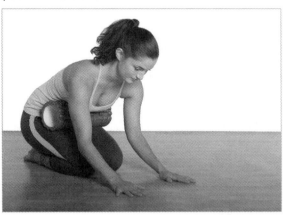

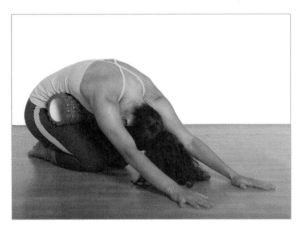

Lower Back Stretch

Starting Position: While kneeling, place the roller across your thighs at the hip crease. Place a rolled-up towel under your knees for comfort, if desired.

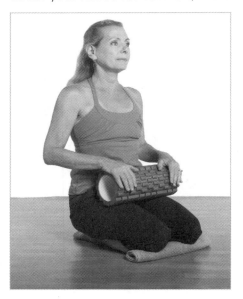

1: Lower your butt to your heels and walk your hands forward along the ground, until your arms are extended. You'll notice a stretch in your upper and lower back. Hold as tolerated. Breathe slowly and fully. As your muscles relax, tuck your chin to your chest and extend your reach to increase the stretch. Try to keep your butt as close to your heels as possible.

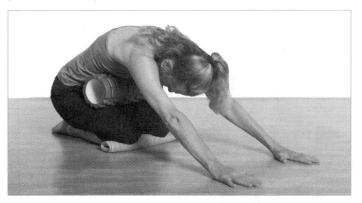

Chest Release

Starting Position: With the roller either positioned vertically or horizontally, carefully lie facedown on the roller; your toes should rest on the ground. Extend your arms out to the sides in a "T."

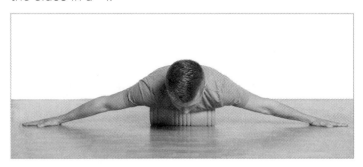

1: Keeping your abs tight, slowly lift your arms a few inches off the floor. Hold.

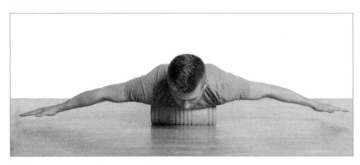

Return to starting position.

Chest & Shoulder Release

Caution: Do not apply too much pressure as this can cut off circulation to the area.

The Position: Lie facedown with your right arm extended to the side and your left arm in a comfortable location (maybe under your face) to offer support. Place the roller parallel to your body at the intersection of your right shoulder joint and chest. Apply gentle pressure into the roller. Hold for 5 seconds, no longer. Breathe slowly and fully.

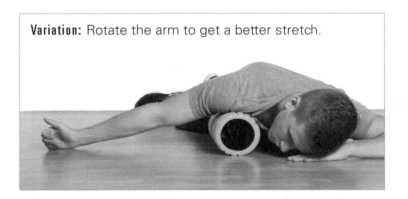

Variation: Rotate the arm to get a better stretch.

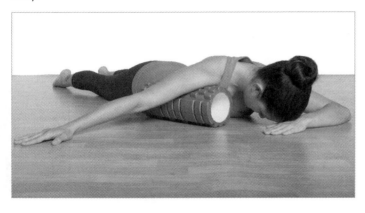

Repeat on the opposite arm.

Biceps Release

You may want to place a pillow under you if you're bony.

Starting Position: Lie facedown with your right arm extended to the side and your left arm in a comfortable location (maybe under your face) to offer support. Place the roller at the top of your right biceps.

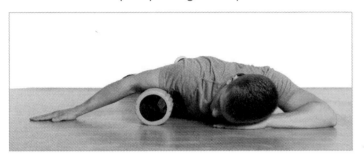

1: Apply gentle pressure into the roller. Hold for a few seconds. Roll your body slowly to roll the roller along your biceps. Apply static pressure as needed to address any tight spots. Hold as tolerated. Breathe slowly and fully.

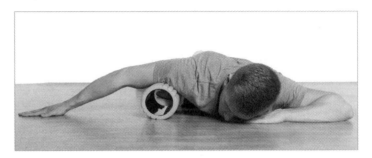

Repeat on the opposite arm.

Hip Flexor Release

The Position: Lie facedown, resting on your forearms for support. Carefully position the roller at your hip crease. Hold for 5 seconds, breathing slowly and fully.

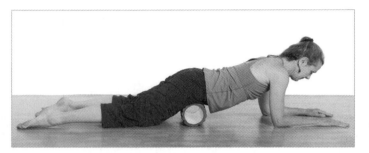

Variation: To increase pressure, don't lean on your forearms; just lie flat while allowing your hips to press into the roller.

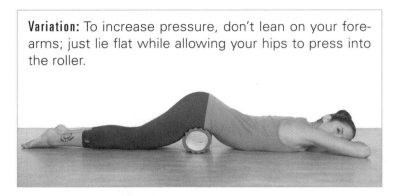

Quad Release

The Position: Lie facedown, resting on your forearms for support. Place a rolled-up towel under your knees for comfort, if desired. Carefully position the roller across your thighs. Hold for 5 seconds, breathing slowly and fully.

Variation: To increase pressure, don't lean on your forearms; just lie flat while allowing your hips to press into the roller.

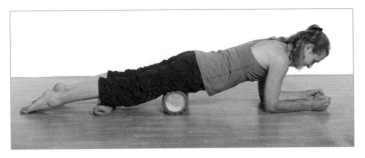

Reposition the roller further down your thigh, either by moving your body with your arms or manually positioning the roller with your hands, and repeat.

Spine Extension

Caution: Avoid this exercise if you have lower back issues.

Starting Position: Lie on your stomach with your arms extended above your head, forearms resting on a roller with your palms facing each other. Your legs are straight behind you and your head is slightly off the ground with eyes looking down.

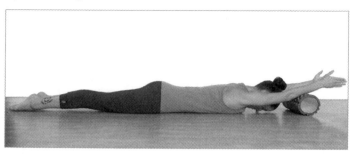

1: Slowly inhale as you roll the roller toward you, pulling your shoulder blades down. Let your head, chest and upper back rise.

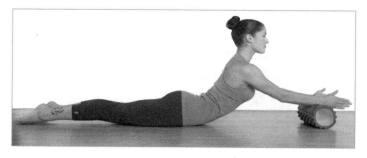

Slowly exhale as you reverse the movement.

Glute Massage

Starting Position: Sit on a roller that's either placed horizontally on the floor or a chair. Shift your weight so that you're on one butt cheek.

1: Slowly roll your rear end forward then backward, stopping at any point along the way that requires a little more attention.

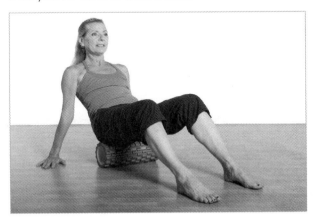

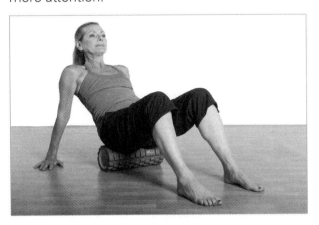

Variation: Slowly lean to the left and hold, and then shift your weight to the right.

Advanced Variation: Place your right ankle on top of your left knee and perform the massage. Remember to switch sides.

Upper Back Release

Starting Position: Lie on your back with your knees bent and feet flat on the floor. Place the roller under your shoulder blades and then reach your arms toward the ceiling.

1–2: Use your legs to slowly move your body up and down the roller, stopping along the way to focus on any tight spots. Breathe slowly and fully.

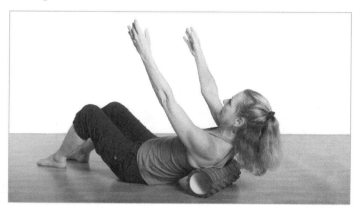

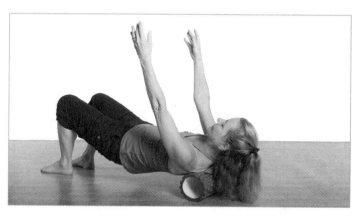

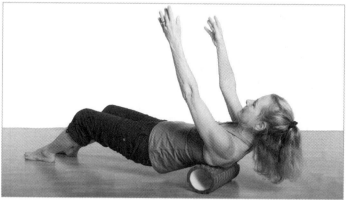

Variation: Depending on how much stretch you want/need, you can also support your head with your hands or reach your arms by your ears.

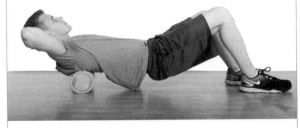

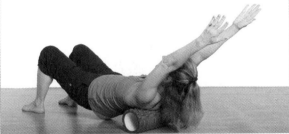

Upper Back & Shoulder Massage

This exercise challenges your core as well as releases your shoulders and back.

Starting Position: Place a roller on the floor and lie on it from head to tailbone. Place your feet on the floor, with your knees bent and arms out to the side for additional stability. Once stable, raise your arms directly above your chest.

1–2: Slowly move your body left and right; try not to fall off the roller.

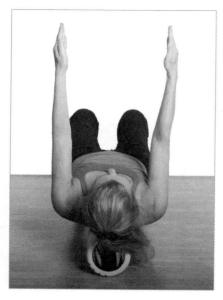

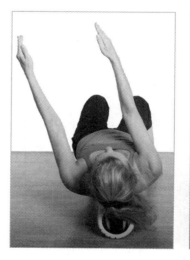

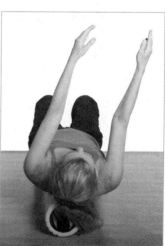

Modification: You can keep your arms on the floor for support.

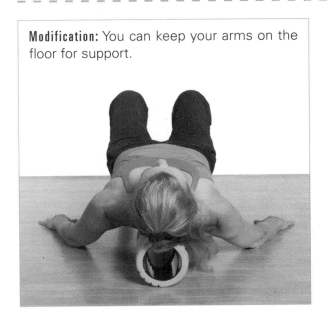

Variation: You can also cross your arms across your chest.

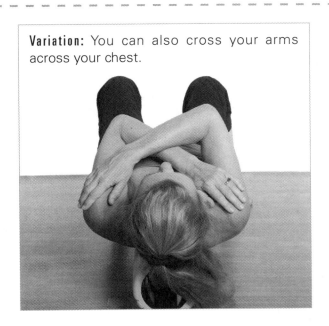

Neck Release

Caution: Avoid this move if you have neck issues, impaired circulation in the neck area or skeletal concerns.

Starting Position: Lie on your back with your knees bent and feet flat on the floor. Position the roller the under your neck. Slowly breathe in through your nose and out through your mouth as you allow your back to settle and relax.

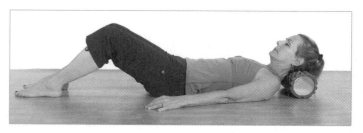

1–2: Once tension is released, gently turn your head left and then right. Use small, slow movements. Listen to your body. Hold for 5 to 30 seconds.

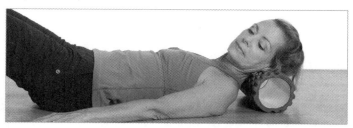

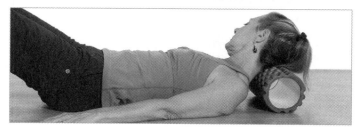

Variation: Straighten your legs to increase the downward pressure on the neck.

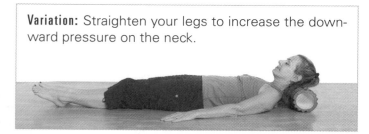

Chest Expander

This exercise is designed to open up your rib cage and allow better breathing.

Starting Position: Place a roller on the floor and lie on it from head to tailbone. Place your feet on the floor, with your knees bent and arms out to the side for additional stability. Once stable, raise your arms directly above your chest.

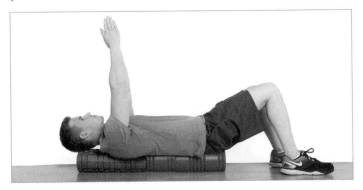

1: Slowly move one arm forward and the other back as you breathe in through your nose and out through pursed lips.

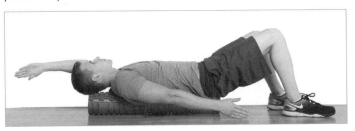

2: Switch arms and continue switching while focusing on mindful breathing and rib cage expansion.

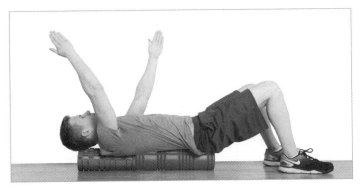

Shoulders & Hips Challenge

Starting Position: Place a roller on the floor and lie on it from head to tailbone. Place your feet on the floor, with your knees bent and arms out to the side for additional stability. Once stable, raise your arms directly above your chest.

1: Keeping your legs together throughout the exercise, lower your right arm by your ear and extend your left leg.

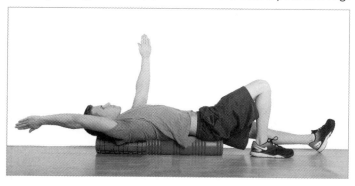

Return to starting position. Repeat on the other side, maintaining proper form and posture.

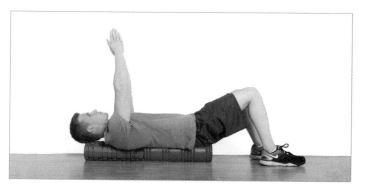

Mid-Back Release

The Position: Lie on the roller so that it's under your spine from your tailbone to your neck. Bend your knees and place your feet flat on the floor. Extend your arms out to the sides along the floor into a "T" position. Hold for 5 to 30 seconds. Breathe slowly and fully.

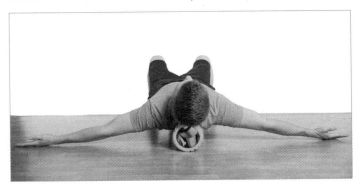

Modification: To challenge your core, reach your arms up to the ceiling. You can also straighten your legs to increase the pressure, as well as roll left and right.

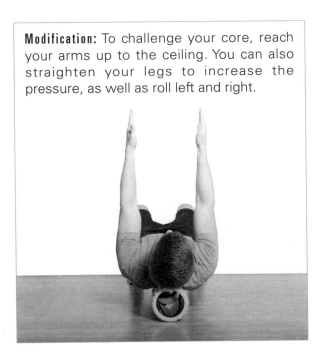

Lower Back Expansion

Caution: Take care if you have facet lower back issues.

The Position: Lie on your back with your knees bent and feet flat on the floor. Place the roller directly under your lower back. Gently press your lower back into the roller and hold for 5 to 30 seconds. Breathe slowly and deeply.

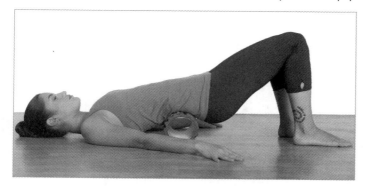

Supine Fly

Caution: Do not do this is exercise if you have shoulder problems.

Starting Position: Place a roller on the floor and lie on it from head to tailbone. Place your feet on the floor, with your knees bent and your arms on the floor. Once stable, bring your hands above your chest.

1: Slowly spread your arms out to the side; hold and relax, feeling the stretch.

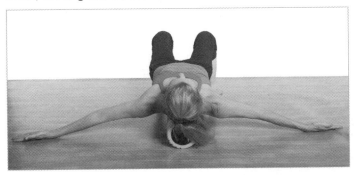

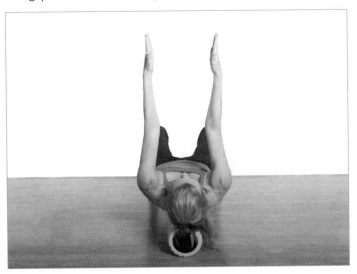

Modification: You don't have to open up your arms all the way.

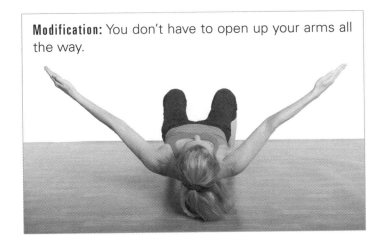

Shoulder Protraction/Retraction

Starting Position: Place a roller on the floor and lie on it from head to tailbone. Place your feet on the floor, with your knees bent and your arms on the floor. Once stable, bring your hands together above your chest.

1: Maintaining neutral spine, exhale and broaden your upper back to reach your fingertips to the ceiling. Hold.

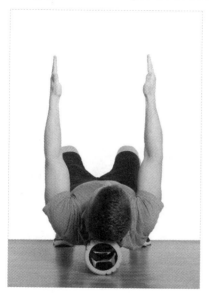

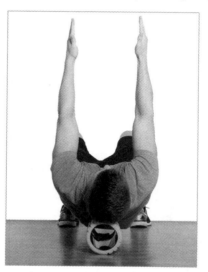

Inhale and gently return your shoulder blades to starting position.

Hip Flexor Extender

Starting Position: Lie on your back with your knees bent and feet flat on the floor. Place the roller directly under your lower back.

1: Gently press your lower back into the roller and hold for 5 to 30 seconds. Breathe slowly and deeply. Then grab under your right thigh and gently pull your knee to your chest as you extend your left leg to the floor. Hold.

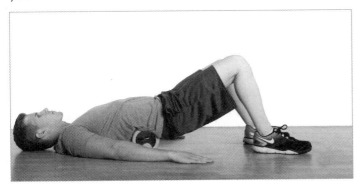

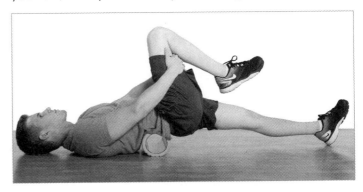

Switch legs.

Modification: If flexibility is an issue, lie on the roller from head to tailbone.

Supine I's, Y's & T's

Note: This exercise has three levels. Be sure to attain perfect form before moving on to the next level.

Starting Position: Place a roller on the floor and lie on it from head to tailbone. Place your feet on the floor, with your knees bent and your arms extended toward the ceiling, palms facing each other.

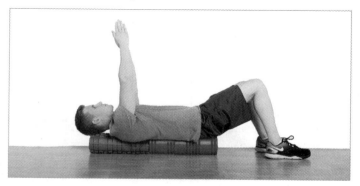

Level 1 (I's)

1: Keeping your arms straight, slowly move both arms back toward the floor, leading with your thumbs. Your body will look like an "I" from a bird's-eye view.

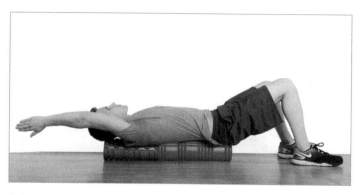

Return to starting position and repeat the "I" position as desired before moving on to the next level.

Level 2 (Y's)

1: Leading with your thumbs, move both arms back toward the floor and slightly out to the sides in order to make a "Y."

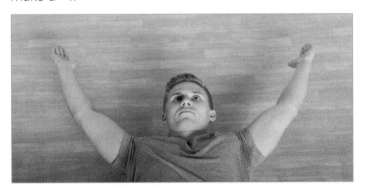

Return to starting position and repeat the "Y" position as desired before moving on to the next level.

Level 3 (T's)

1: Spread your arms wide apart and drop your knuckles to the floor to make a "T."

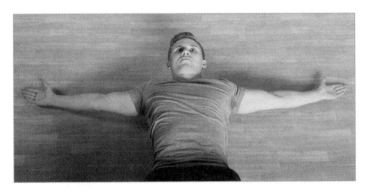

Return to starting position and repeat the "T" position as desired.

Supine Marching

Starting Position: Place a roller on the floor and lie on it from head to tailbone. Place your feet on the floor, with your knees bent and hands along your sides.

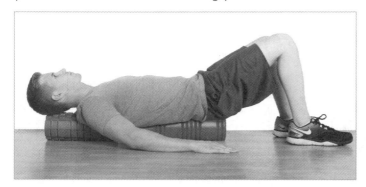

1: Once stable, slowly lift your left foot slightly off the floor (the less you lift your foot off the floor, the more challenging this exercise is). Hold this position for 5 to 15 seconds, making sure you maintain proper alignment. Do not allow your torso or hips to rock.

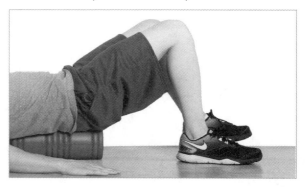

2: Return to starting position and switch sides.

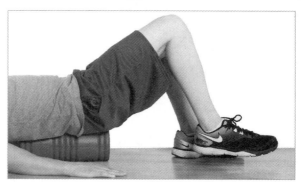

Total Calf Release

This can be performed on one or both calves at the same time.

Starting Position: Sit with your legs extended, propping yourself up on your elbows and/or hands. Place the roller at the top of your calf muscle near the knee.

1: Using your arms to move your legs, slowly roll the roller up and down the backs of your calves. Hold at tender locations as needed.

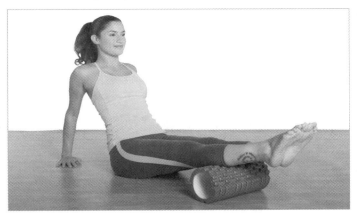

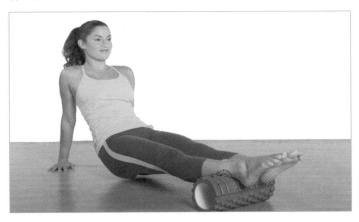

Switch sides.

Modification: This can also be done while lying faceup.

Variation: You can also turn your foot inward and outward to get the inside and outside of the calf.

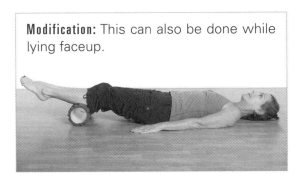

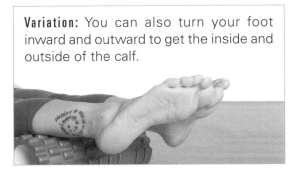

Hamstring Release

This can be performed on one or both hamstrings at the same time.

Starting Position: Sit on the floor with your legs extended and position the roller under your hamstrings closest to the buttock area. You may prop yourself up with your hands to allow for easier rolling of the roller.

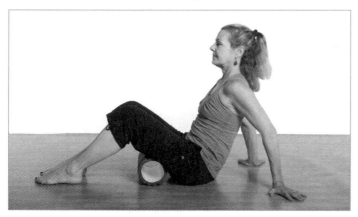

1: Applying the appropriate amount of pressure, manually move or roll the roller up and down your leg. Hold at tender locations as needed. Breathe slowly and fully.

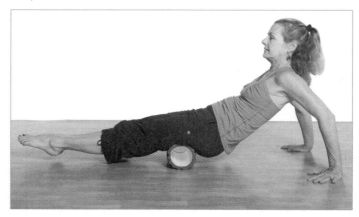

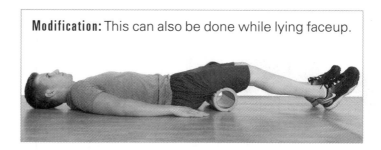

Modification: This can also be done while lying faceup.

Psoas Release

Starting Position: Lie on your back with your knees bent and feet flat on the floor. Place the roller directly under your tailbone.

1: Keeping your left leg in place, hug your right knee to your chest, feeling the stretch in your left leg. You can straighten that leg to intensify the stretch.

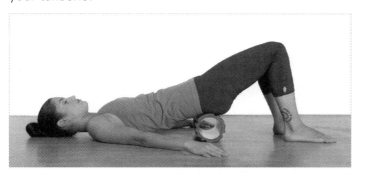

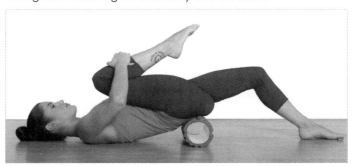

Variation: Rather than keeping the other leg on the ground, you can extend it forward.

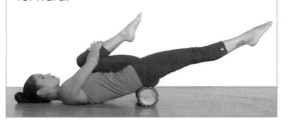

Sacrum Release

The Position: Lie on your back with your knees bent and feet flat on the floor. Position the roller under your tailbone/sacrum and then hug your knees to your chest. Let your weight settle on the roller. If you desire, you can gently shift your weight from side to side.

Variation: This can also be done with your arms along the ground.

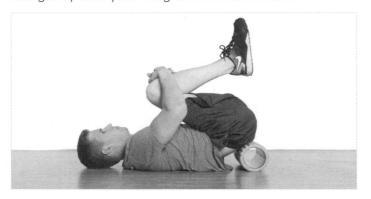

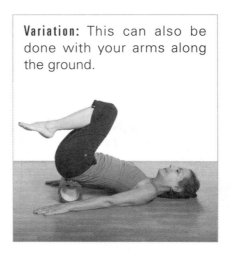

Iliotibial Band Release

Starting Position: Lie on one side and place a roller under your bottom leg. Use your hands and other foot for support.

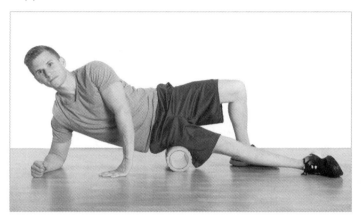

1: Starting just below the hip bone, slowly roll the roller toward but stopping just above the knee. Breathe slowly and fully.

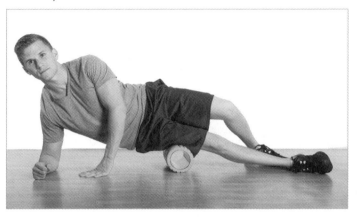

Slowly roll the roller back up to the starting position, stopping at spots along the way that require more attention.

Switch sides.

Piriformis Release

The Position: Sit on the floor and place the roller under your right buttock. Shift your weight to the outer region of your butt. Apply the desired pressure by using your arms to adjust your weight. Press for 5 to 30 seconds. Breathe slowly and fully.

Modification: You can also place your right ankle on your left thigh to focus more on the muscle.

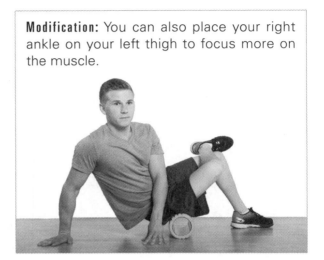

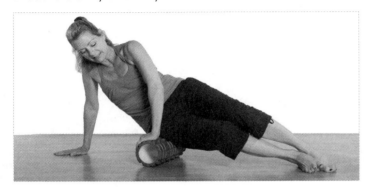

Reposition the roller as necessary. Switch sides.

Lat Release

Caution: Do not roll the roller over your ribs. Avoid this move if you have ribcage or bone-density issues.

Starting Position: Lie on your left side and extend your left arm straight up along the floor. Place a roller just below your armpit.

1: Apply the desired pressure. Press for 5 to 30 seconds, breathing slowly and fully, then slowly roll your body up and down along the roller.

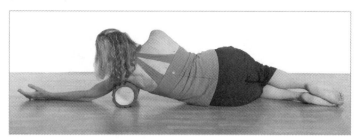

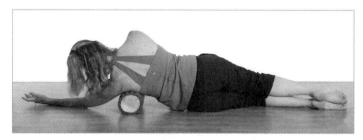

Switch sides.

Triceps Massage

Starting Position: Lie on your right side with your right arm out to the side, palm up. Position the roller alongside your body, under the rear portion of your right arm/triceps, near the shoulder joint. Your arm can be bent or straight.

1: Gently roll the roller up and down the back of your arm, applying the desired pressure. Hold where needed. Breathe fully.

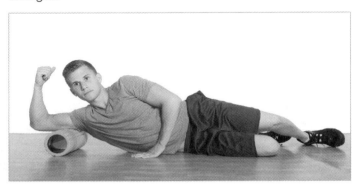

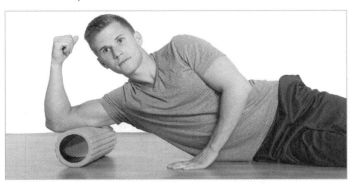

Switch arms.

Waistline Release

Caution: Do not roll the roller over your ribs. Avoid this move if you have ribcage or bone-density issues.

The Position: Lie on your left side and position the roller just above your left hip bone. Apply the desired pressure. Press for 5 to 30 seconds, breathing slowly and fully. Then lower your left shoulder toward the floor to increase the stretch.

Variation: Extend your top arm over your head until it's parallel with the floor.

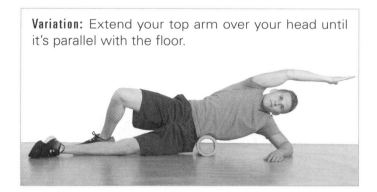

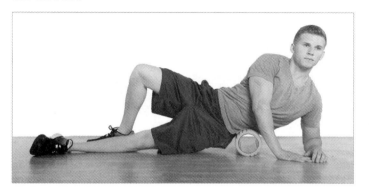

Switch sides.

Inner Thigh Massage

Starting Position: Lie on your left side and position the roller between your thighs; you can keep your legs straight or slightly bent. You can rest your head on your left arm or prop your head up with your hand.

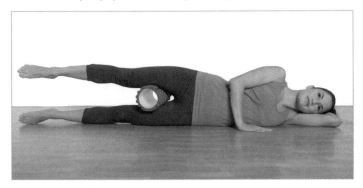

1: Squeeze your thighs into the roller for 5 to 30 seconds. Breathe slowly and fully.

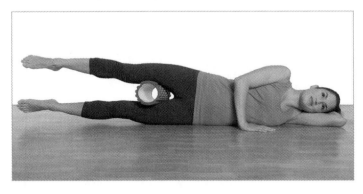

Reposition the roller as necessary. Switch sides.

Variation: Keeping the lower leg on the floor, press the top thigh into the roller.

Combo Special

You may need several rollers to enjoy this one. Also, you may need a helper to place all the rollers in the correct location.

The Position: Dim the lights, turn on relaxing music, turn off all distractions and then lie on your back. Place one roller under your calves or hamstrings, and one under your neck. Just be—relax and turn off all your concerns for as long as you can. If it's easier, tense a muscle for 5 seconds, and then exhale and breathe. Aim for 5 to 10 minutes.

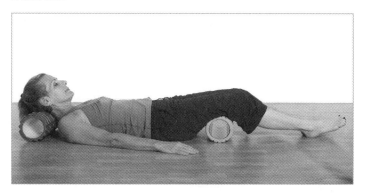

Index

Acknowledgments

My sincere appreciation goes out to Lily Chou and Claire Chun of the Ulysses Press editorial team for their superior professionalism. A special thanks goes out to photographer Austin Forbord of Rapt Productions and models Christopher Caruthers, Toni Silver and Nadia Velasquez for their patience. I'd also like to thank Chris Knopf and the others who shared their practical knowledge about trigger point treatments. Thanks to my wife Margaret of 36 years for her support, and finally a shout out to Kevin Knopf as a winner on the Price Is Right. Lastly, many thanks to the administrators at Ulysses Press for allowing me the opportunity to write for them.

About the Author

Karl Knopf, has authored numerous books (including *Foam Roller Workbook*, *Therapy Ball Workbook*, *Healthy Hips Handbook*, *Healthy Shoulder Handbook*, *Stretching for 50+*, *Weights for 50+* and *Total Sports Conditioning for Athletes 50+*) that present safe and sane ways to improve the fitness of adults of all levels and ages. During his 40 years of teaching, he has served in many capacities with the fitness industry, from consultant on National Institutes of Health grants to advisor to the series Sit and Be Fit and to the State of California on disability issues. He has even worked with large health insurance companies to bring fitness programs to their members. Knopf has been featured in the *Wall Street Journal* and other national publications. He is retired from Foothill College in Los Altos, California, where he taught adaptive fitness classes and directed the fitness therapy program. Knopf now serves as a director of fitness therapy and senior fitness programs for the International Sports Science Association. Dr. Karl, as his students like to call him, was recently selected to the Health Advisory Board for Santa Clara County as an advisor to San Jose State University's Human Performance Department.